# The Hashimoto's Diet Cookbook

## Easy and Tasty Recipes to Promote Wellness and Reverse Hypothyroid

**Lourdes Harkins**

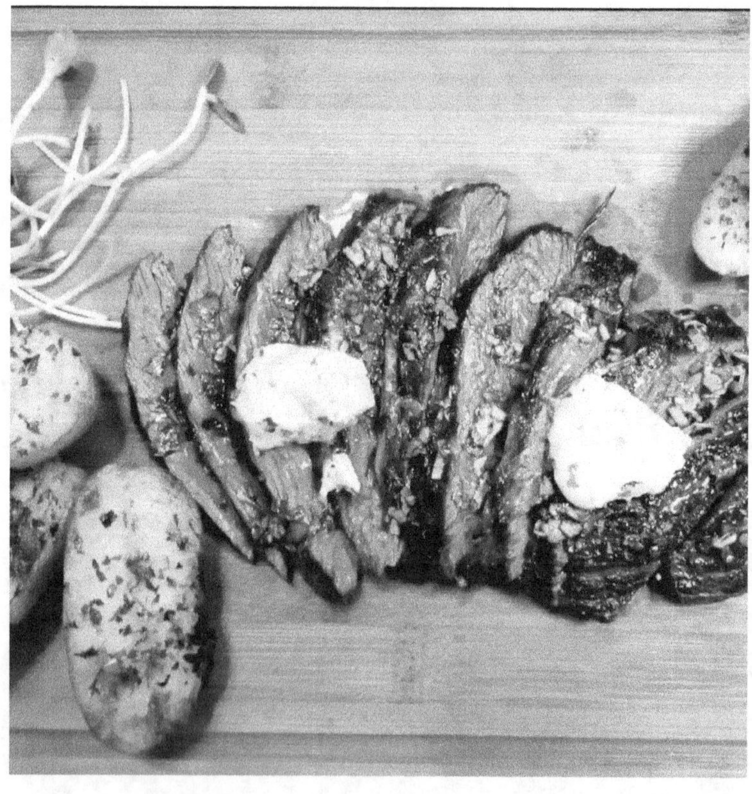

# Table of Content

# INTRODUCTION

John, a 35-year-old man, had been struggling with the symptoms of Hashimoto's disease for years. Fatigue, weight gain, and a general feeling of sluggishness had become his daily companions. Frustrated with the lack of progress from medication alone, he decided to explore other options.

After extensive research, John discovered that diet could play a significant role in managing Hashimoto's. He adopted a gluten-free and dairy-free diet, focusing on nutrient-dense foods like fruits, vegetables, lean proteins, and healthy fats. He also incorporated stress-reducing activities such as yoga and meditation into his routine.

Within a few weeks, John noticed a remarkable improvement in his symptoms. His energy levels surged, and the excess weight began to melt away. The brain fog lifted, and he felt more focused and clear-headed.

John's success story inspired him to share his experience with others. He started a blog to raise awareness about the connection between diet and Hashimoto's disease, offering tips and recipes to help fellow sufferers.

Through his dedication to a healthier lifestyle and mindful eating, John regained control of his life. He learned that with a well-balanced diet and self-care, even in the face of an autoimmune condition like Hashimoto's, he could find renewed vitality and happiness.

Hashimoto's disease, often known as Hashimoto's thyroiditis, is a chronic autoimmune thyroid illness. It is the most prevalent cause of hypothyroidism (underactive thyroid) in the United States and many other nations and is named after the Japanese physician Hakaru Hashimoto, who first diagnosed the condition in 1912.

The immune system wrongly assaults the thyroid gland in Hashimoto's disease, causing inflammation and damage.

The thyroid gland, which is positioned in the front of the neck, generates hormones that govern a variety of biological activities such as metabolism, growth, and energy levels. When the immune system attacks the thyroid, it gradually reduces its capacity to create enough thyroid hormones.

Hashimoto's disease develops slowly and may go undiagnosed in its early stages. It typically affects middle-aged women, although it can afflict males of all ages, including youngsters.

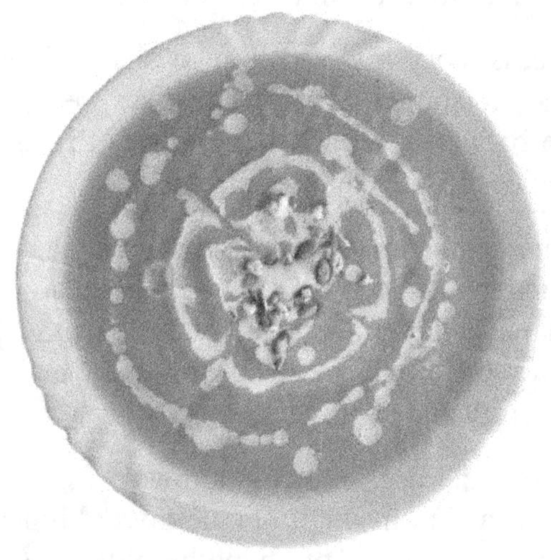

# CAUSES OF HASHIMOTO'S

Although the roots of Hashimoto's illness are unknown, experts believe it is caused by a mix of genetic and environmental variables.

**Genetic Factors:** There is evidence that some genes have a role in predisposing people to Hashimoto's illness. A family history of autoimmune disorders, particularly thyroid-related problems, raises the likelihood of getting Hashimoto's. This suggests that there may be particular genetic variants that contribute to the disease's development.

**Environmental variables:** It is considered that a variety of environmental variables cause or contribute to the development of Hashimoto's disease. Among the possible factors are:

**Hormonal Changes:** Hormonal changes such as those experienced during puberty, pregnancy, or menopause may alter the immune system's response and contribute to the development of Hashimoto's disease.

**Infections:** Certain viral or bacterial infections have been proposed as possible Hashimoto's disease causes. These illnesses may cause an inappropriate immunological response to the thyroid gland.

**Iodine Levels:** Adequate iodine levels are required for thyroid hormone synthesis. Iodine shortage and high iodine consumption have both been associated the development of Hashimoto's disease, while the relationship is complicated and varies depending on individual circumstances.

**Other Autoimmune disorders:** People who have other autoimmune disorders, such as type 1 diabetes, rheumatoid arthritis, or lupus, are more likely to acquire Hashimoto's disease. This shows that diverse autoimmune illnesses may share underlying mechanisms or genetic predispositions.

It is crucial to note that, while these variables are thought to contribute to the development of Hashimoto's disease, not everyone who is exposed to them will get the illness. The interaction between genetic vulnerability and environmental stimuli is currently poorly understood and is a topic of continuing research.

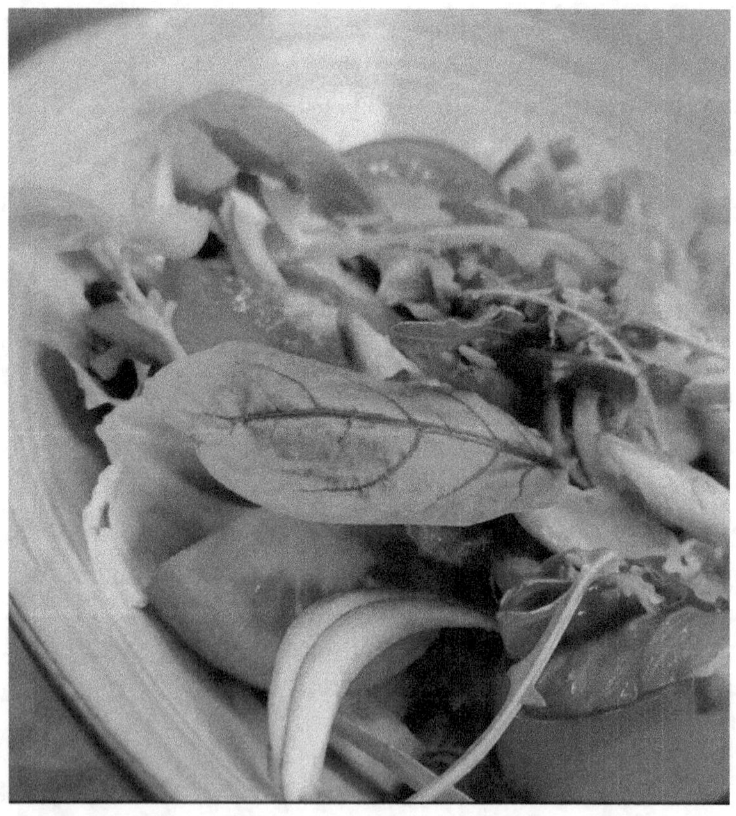

# SYMPTOMS OF HASHIMOTO'S

Hashimoto's illness can induce a wide range of symptoms, the severity of which varies from person to person. Common Hashimoto's symptoms include:

**Weariness and sluggishness:** Many people with Hashimoto's disease report chronic weariness and a lack of vitality. Even after receiving adequate sleep, they may remain fatigued or find it difficult to engage in everyday activities.

**Weight Gain or Difficulties Shedding Weight:** Hashimoto's can cause the body's metabolism to slow down, resulting in weight gain or difficulties shedding weight. This may be accompanied by increased fluid retention and bloating.

**Cold Sensitivity:** People with Hashimoto's may be more sensitive to cold temperatures. They may feel cold even when others are warm, and they may have icy hands and feet.

**Dry Skin and Hair:** The condition can result in dry, rough, and itchy skin. Hair might become dry, brittle, and brittle. Some people may also notice thinning of the brows.

**Muscle Weakness or Stiffness:** Muscle weakness, pains, or stiffness can be caused by Hashimoto's disease. This might take the form of overall muscular tiredness or particular joint and muscle problems.

**Constipation:** An underactive thyroid can cause the digestive system to slow down, resulting in constipation and trouble passing feces.

**Depression or Mood Swings:** Hashimoto's can have an impact on mood and mental health. People may suffer sadness, irritation, anxiety, or mood changes.

**Memory Issues or Brain Fog:** Some patients with Hashimoto's disease report difficulty concentrating, recalling memories, and thinking clearly. This is commonly referred to as "brain fog."

**Menstrual Irregularities in Women:** Women with Hashimoto's disease may suffer changes in their menstrual cycle, such as heavier or irregular periods.

**Thyroid Gland Swelling (Goiter):** Hashimoto's illness can cause the thyroid gland to grow in certain cases, resulting in a visible or palpable swelling in the front of the neck known as a goiter.

It's important to note that not everyone with Hashimoto's disease will have all of these symptoms, and the intensity and mix of symptoms might vary across people. If you believe you have Hashimoto's disease or are experiencing any of these symptoms, you should see a doctor for an accurate diagnosis and proper treatment.

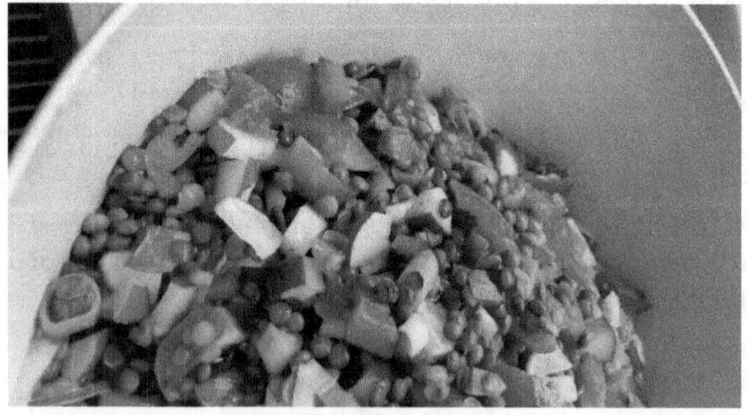

# TIPS TO TREAT HASHIMOTO'S

*Here are some suggestions for dealing with Hashimoto's:*

**Prescription and Regular Monitoring:** To manage thyroid hormone levels, follow your healthcare provider's prescription schedule. Thyroid hormone levels must be monitored regularly to ensure appropriate therapy and, if necessary, medication dose adjustments.

**Diet and Nutrition:** Consider eating a well-balanced diet rich in nutrient-dense foods. Lean proteins, fruits and vegetables, healthy fats, and gluten-free whole grains are examples of such foods.

Some people with Hashimoto's disease find that reducing gluten and/or dairy from their diet helps them feel better. To create a tailored food plan, consult with a qualified nutritionist.

**Stress management:** Chronic stress can have a deleterious influence on the immune system and thyroid function. Participate in stress-relieving activities such as meditation, deep breathing exercises, yoga, or other relaxation techniques that suit you.

**Regular Physical Activity:** Include regular physical activity in your routine since it can assist enhance your energy levels, mood, and general well-being. Select activities that you love and check with your healthcare practitioner to identify the best fitness alternatives for you.

**Sleep and Rest:** Make proper sleep and rest a priority to enhance overall health and thyroid function. To encourage excellent rest, aim for a consistent sleep schedule and establish a sleep-friendly atmosphere.

**Supplements:** Check with your healthcare physician to see whether certain supplements are right for you. Selenium, vitamin D, omega-3 fatty acids, and probiotics are common supplements for people with Hashimoto's disease. Individual requirements and proper doses may vary, thus expert advice is essential.

**Mind-Body Practices:** Consider adding mind-body practices such as mindfulness meditation, relaxation methods, or emotional well-being activities. These can aid in stress reduction, immune function support, and general quality of life.

**Support Network:** Seek aid from friends, family, or support groups to cope with the mental and physical issues that might accompany Hashimoto's disease management. Sharing your experiences and expertise with other people who have the illness can give useful support and insights.

Remember that everyone's experience with Hashimoto's is unique, and treatment techniques may differ. Working together with your healthcare team to build a tailored treatment plan that meets your unique needs and concerns is critical.

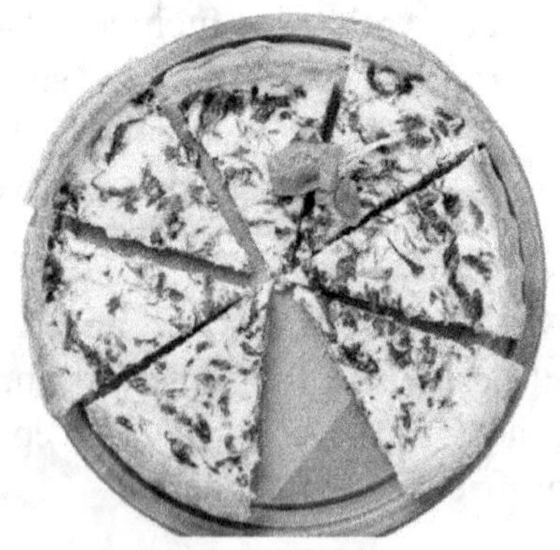

# THE RECIPES

# BREAKFAST

## *Veggie Omelet*

### Ingredients

- 2-3 whole eggs or egg whites
- Various vegetables:
- 1/2 cup spinach, chopped
- 1/4 cup bell peppers, chopped
- 1/4 cup mushrooms, sliced
- 2 tbsp. finely chopped onions
- Season with salt and pepper to taste.
- Herbs of Provence (optional)

### Instructions

In a mixing bowl, whisk together the eggs or egg whites and season with salt and pepper.

Heat a tiny quantity of oil or frying spray in a nonstick skillet over medium heat.

Sauté the veggies in the pan until they are slightly softened.

Pour the beaten eggs over the veggies and heat until the edges begin to set.

Fold the omelet in half gently and cook for a few minutes more, or until thoroughly done.

If preferred, garnish with fresh herbs and serve warm.

# *Overnight Gluten-Free Chia Pudding*

## Ingredients

- 2 tbsp of chia seeds
- 1 cup milk substitute (almond, coconut, etc.)
- 1-2 tablespoons honey or maple syrup

## Flavorings to choose from

- A half teaspoon of vanilla extract
- A quarter teaspoon of cinnamon

**Toppings:** berries and nuts

## Instructions

Combine chia seeds, dairy-free milk, sweetener, and flavorings in a jar or container.

Stir everything up thoroughly and place in the fridge overnight or for at least a few hours.

Give it a thorough swirl before serving to ensure the chia seeds are well dispersed and have absorbed the liquid.

Garnish with your favorite fresh berries and almonds.

# Quinoa Breakfast Bowl

## Ingredients

- 1 cooked cup of quinoa
- Fruit slices: 1/2 banana
- A quarter cup of berries

## Optional garnishes

- 1 tbsp almond butter
- 1 tbsp. seeds or nuts

## Instructions

Cook quinoa according to package directions, adding water or milk for creaminess if desired.

Transfer the cooked quinoa to a bowl.

Top with your favorite sliced fruits.

Sprinkle with seeds or nuts and drizzle with nut butter.

Stir gently to blend, then serve.

# Smoothie Bowl

## Ingredients

- 1 frozen fruit cup:
- A half-cup of berries
- 1 mango cup
- A handful of leafy greens (spinach, kale, and so on)

## Your favorite liquid:

- A half-cup almond milk
- Coconut water, for example.

**Toppings:**

- 2 granola tablespoons
- 1 tbsp. shredded coconut
- 1 tbsp almond butter

## Instructions

Blend the frozen fruits, leafy greens, and liquid in a blender.

Blend until the mixture is smooth and creamy. Adjust the liquid amount to get the appropriate consistency.

Fill a bowl halfway with the smoothie.

Top with granola, shredded coconut, a dollop of nut butter, or any toppings you choose.

Serve with a spoon.

## *Avocado Toast*

### Ingredients

- 2 slices toasted gluten-free bread
- Avocado, ripe (1/2 to 1 entire, depending on size)
- To taste, sea salt

### Optional garnishes

- Tomato slices
- 1 boiled egg
- Microgreens

### Instructions

Toast the gluten-free bread until it is golden brown.

Remove the pit from the avocado and scoop out the flesh.

With a fork, mash the avocado and distribute it on the toasted bread.

Season with sea salt.

Toppings such as sliced tomatoes, a poached egg, or microgreens are optional.

Serve immediately and enjoy.

## *Yogurt Parfait*

### Ingredients

- 1 cup vegan yogurt (coconut, almond, etc.)
- 1/2 cup strawberries, mixed berries
- Blueberries, raspberries, and so on.
- (1/4 cup) gluten-free granola

**Optional:** honey or maple syrup

Optional seeds (chia, flax, etc.) for sprinkling

### Instructions

Layer dairy-free yogurt in a glass or a dish.

On top of the yogurt, put a layer of mixed berries.

Sprinkle gluten-free granola on top of the berries.

Repeat the layers until you achieve the required quantity.

If desired, drizzle with honey or maple syrup.

To add texture and nutrients, sprinkle with seeds.

Enjoy!

## *Sweet Potato Hash*

### Ingredients

- 1 cup chopped sweet potatoes
- 1/4 cup finely chopped onions
- 1/4 cup bell peppers, sliced

### Protein of preference:

- 1/4 cup chicken, turkey sausage, etc.
- Spices and herbs:
- Paprika, 1/2 teaspoon
- A quarter teaspoon of cumin
- A quarter teaspoon of rosemary
- Season with salt and pepper to taste.

### Instructions

Heat a tiny quantity of oil or frying spray in a pan over medium heat.

Cook the diced sweet potatoes in the pan until they begin to soften.

In the skillet, combine the chopped onions, sliced bell peppers, and protein of choice.

Cook until the sweet potatoes are tender and the onions are transparent.

Season with herbs, spices, salt, and pepper to taste.

Stir everything together thoroughly.

As a delicious hash, serve warm.

## *Buckwheat Pancakes*

### Ingredients

- 1 buckwheat flour cup
- 1 tbsp coconut sugar or your preferred sweetener
- 1 tsp. baking powder
- 1 teaspoon salt
- 1 cup milk substitute (almond, coconut, etc.)
- 1 tbsp melted coconut oil or other oil of choice

### Optional garnishes

- Fruits that are in season
- Yogurt made without dairy
- Maple syrup, for example.

### Instructions

In a mixing dish, combine buckwheat flour, coconut sugar, baking powder, and salt.

Combine the dry ingredients with dairy-free milk and melted coconut oil.

Stir until smooth and completely blended.

Melt butter in a nonstick pan or griddle over medium heat.

For each pancake, pour 1/4 cup batter into the skillet.

Cook until bubbles appear on the surface, then turn and cook until golden on the other side.

Repeat with the rest of the batter.

Enjoy the pancakes with your favorite toppings!

## *Vegetable Frittata*

### Ingredients

- 4-5 eggs (egg whites or whole eggs)

### Various vegetables:

- 1/2 cup thinly chopped zucchini
- 1 cup spinach, packed
- 1 pound cherry tomatoes

Season with salt and pepper to taste.

Herbs of Provence (optional)

### Instructions

Preheat the oven to 375 degrees F (190 degrees C).

Sauté the veggies in an oven-safe pan until they are slightly softened.

In a mixing bowl, whisk together the eggs or egg whites and season with salt and pepper.

Pour the beaten eggs over the skillet's sautéed veggies.

Cook until the edges begin to firm on the stovetop over medium heat.

Bake for around 10-15 minutes, or until the frittata is thoroughly cooked and slightly brown on top, in a preheated oven.

If desired, garnish with fresh herbs.

Allow it to cool somewhat before slicing and serving.

## *Green Smoothie*

### Ingredients

- A handful of leafy greens (spinach, kale, and so on)

### Fruit salad:

- A half banana
- 1 pound pineapple chunks
- 1/2 apple

### Your favorite liquid:

- 1 cup of coconut water or
- Almond milk, for example.

Protein powder or nut butter are optional for extra protein.

**Optional:** .ice cubes

### Instructions

Blend the leafy greens, mixed fruits, drink, and optional protein powder or nut butter in a blender.

Blend until the mixture is smooth and creamy. If desired, add ice cubes.

Fill a glass or bowl halfway with the smoothie.

Serve it as a light and nutritious breakfast.

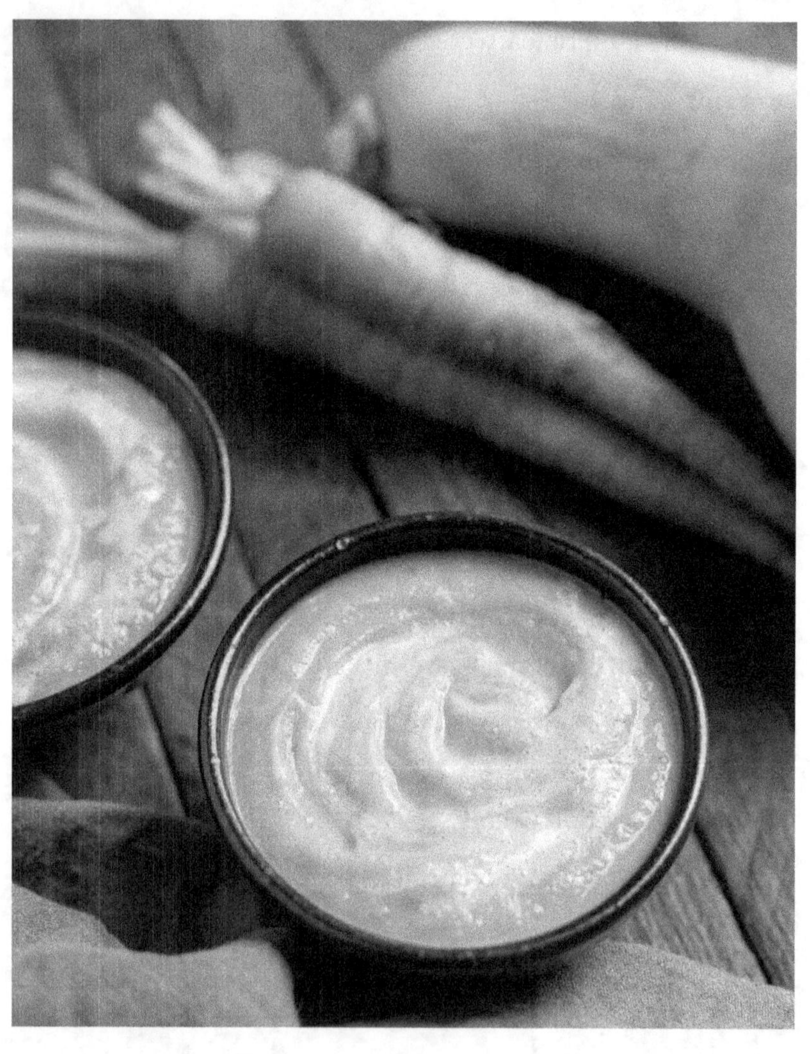

# LUNCH RECIPES

## *Salad with Quinoa*

### Ingredients

- 1 cup quinoa, cooked
- 1/2 cup chopped cucumber, mixed veggies
- 1/2 cup cherry tomatoes, halved
- 1/4 cup bell peppers, chopped
- Leafy greens (spinach, arugula, and so forth) - a small number

### Protein of preference

- 4 ounces grilled of chicken
- 12 cup chickpeas
- 4 ounces tofu
- 2 tbsp olive oil for dressing
- 1 teaspoon of lemon juice

Season with salt and pepper to taste.

### Instructions

Combine the cooked quinoa, mixed veggies, leafy greens, and protein of choice in a mixing dish.

To create the dressing, mix the olive oil, lemon juice, salt, and pepper in a separate small bowl.

Toss the quinoa salad with the dressing until evenly coated.

Chill or serve at room temperature.

## Greek Salad

### Ingredients

- Salad greens, mixed - 2 cups
- 1/2 cup chopped cucumbers -
- 1/2 cup halved cherry tomatoes -
- 1/4 cup Kalamata olives
- 2 teaspoons finely sliced red onion
- 1/4 cup crumbled feta cheese

### Dressing:

- 2 tbsp of olive oil
- 1 teaspoon of lemon juice
- A half teaspoon of dried oregano

Season with salt and pepper to taste.

### Instructions

Combine the mixed salad greens, diced cucumbers, halved cherry tomatoes, Kalamata olives, red onion, and crumbled feta cheese in a large mixing basin.

To create the dressing, mix the olive oil, lemon juice, dried oregano, salt, and pepper in a separate small bowl.

Toss the salad lightly with the dressing to mix.

Serve right away.

# *Soup with Lentils*

## Ingredients

- 1 cup lentils, dry
- 1/2 cup diced onion
- 1/2 cup diced carrots
- 1/2 cup diced celery
- 2 cloves minced garlic
- 4 cups vegetable broth

## Spices and herbs

- 1 tablespoon cumin
- Paprika, 1/2 teaspoon
- 1/2 teaspoon fresh thyme

Season with salt and pepper to taste.

## Instructions

Remove any debris from the dry lentils by rinsing them under cold water.

Sauté the chopped onion, carrots, celery, and minced garlic in a large saucepan until softened.

To the saucepan, add the washed lentils, vegetable broth, cumin, paprika, thyme, salt, and pepper.

Bring the mixture to a boil, then lower to low heat and continue to cook for 20-25 minutes, or until the lentils are cooked.

Season with salt and pepper to taste.

Serve immediately.

## *Chickpea Salad Wrap*

### Ingredients

- 1 drained and rinsed can of chickpeas (15 oz.
- 2 teaspoons finely chopped red onion
- 1/4 cup chopped bell peppers
- 1/4 cup diced cucumber
- 2 teaspoons chopped fresh parsley
- Lemon juice - 2 tbsp
- 1 teaspoon olive oil

Season with salt and pepper to taste.

Wrapping with whole grain tortillas or lettuce leaves

### Instructions

Combine the drained and rinsed chickpeas, finely sliced red onion, diced bell peppers, diced cucumber, and fresh parsley in a mixing dish.

In a small mixing bowl, combine the lemon juice, olive oil, salt, and pepper.

Toss the chickpea salad with the dressing to evenly cover the ingredients.

Warm whole-grain tortillas or wrap with lettuce leaves.

Wrap the tortillas or lettuce leaves tightly around the chickpea salad.

Serve immediately or refrigerate until ready to serve.

## *Stir-Fry with Quinoa and Vegetables*

### Ingredients

- 1 cup quinoa, cooked
- Vegetables (broccoli, bell peppers, snow peas, and so forth) - 2 cups
- Sliced garlic - 2 garlic cloves
- Grated ginger - 1 tablespoon
- Tamari (gluten-free soy sauce) or soy sauce - 2 teaspoons
- 1 tablespoon sesame oil

**Optional:** protein sources include tofu, chicken, or shrimp.

### Instructions

In a large pan or wok, heat the sesame oil over medium-high heat.

Sauté the minced garlic and grated ginger in the pan for a minute, or until fragrant.

Stir-fry the mixed veggies in the pan until they are tender-crisp.

Cook until tofu, chicken, or shrimp are cooked through, if preferred.

Drizzle tamari or soy sauce over the cooked quinoa in the pan.

Stir-fry everything for a few minutes, until everything is completely mixed and cooked through.

Serve immediately.

## *Mediterranean Hummus Wrap*

### Ingredients

- Wrap or tortilla made from whole grains
- 14 cup hummus
- 1/4 cup sliced cucumber
- Tomatoes, cut - 1/4 cup
- Pitted and sliced Kalamata olives - 2 teaspoons
- 2 teaspoons finely sliced red onion
- 2 tablespoons crumbled feta cheese
- 1 tablespoon chopped fresh herbs (such as parsley or basil)

### Instructions

Place a clean surface on top of the whole-grain wrap or tortilla.

Spread the hummus evenly throughout the wrap.

In the middle of the wrap, layer cucumber slices, tomato slices, Kalamata olives, red onion slices, crumbled feta cheese, and fresh herbs.

Fold the wrap in half, then roll it firmly from one end to the other.

Serve the wrap cut in half.

## *Veggie Quinoa Buddha Bowl*

### Ingredients

- 1 cup cooked quinoa
- Vegetable mixture (roasted sweet potatoes, steamed broccoli, sautéed mushrooms, and so on).
- Avocado, thinly cut
- Cherry tomatoes,
- Halved radishes
- Chopped fresh herbs (parsley or cilantro)

**Dressing ingredients:** include olive oil, lemon juice, Dijon mustard, salt, and pepper.

### Instructions

Arrange cooked quinoa, mixed veggies, sliced avocado, split cherry tomatoes, and sliced radishes in a mixing bowl.

Garnish with fresh herbs.

To create the dressing, mix the olive oil, lemon juice, Dijon mustard, salt, and pepper in a separate small bowl.

Dress the Buddha bowl with the dressing.

Gently toss to mix.

Serve refrigerated or at room temperature.

## Salmon Baked with Roasted Vegetables

### Ingredients

- 1 piece (4-6 ounces) salmon fillet
- Vegetable mixture (carrots, Brussels sprouts, and cauliflower)
- 1 teaspoon olive oil
- 1 tbsp lemon juice
- Minced garlic - 2 garlic cloves
- Spices and herbs (such as dill, thyme, and paprika)

Season with salt and pepper to taste.

### Instructions

Preheat the oven to 400 degrees F (200 degrees C).

Place the salmon fillet on a baking pan lined with parchment paper.

Combine olive oil, lemon juice, minced garlic, herbs, spices, salt, and pepper in a mixing bowl.

Brush the mixture over the salmon fillet to coat it completely.

Toss the mixed veggies with olive oil, salt, and pepper in a separate bowl.

Arrange the mixed veggies on the baking sheet around the salmon.

Bake for 15-20 minutes, or until the salmon is cooked through and the veggies are soft, in a preheated oven.

Serve immediately.

## *Quinoa Stuffed Zucchini Boats*

- 2 medium-sized zucchini
- Cooked quinoa - 1 cup
- Onion, diced - 1/4 cup
- Garlic, minced - 2 cloves
- 1/4 cup chopped bell pepper
- 1/4 cup sliced tomato 1/4 cup chopped spinach
- Spices and herbs (including oregano, basil, and thyme)

Season with salt and pepper to taste.

**Optional topping:** grated cheese

**Instructions**

Preheat the oven to 375 degrees F (190 degrees C).

Slice the zucchini lengthwise and scoop out the centers to make a hollow "boat" shape.

Sauté the chopped onion, minced garlic, diced bell pepper, and diced tomato in a pan until softened.

Stir together the cooked quinoa and chopped spinach in the pan.

Season with herbs, spices, salt, and pepper to taste.

Fill the zucchini halves with the quinoa mixture.

Sprinkle grated cheese on top of each zucchini boat if desired.

Bake the stuffed zucchini boats for 20-25 minutes, or until the zucchini is tender and the filling is well cooked.

Serve immediately.

## *Mexican Quinoa Bowl*

### Ingredients

- 1 cup cooked quinoa
- Black beans, cooked and drained - 1/2 cup
- Corn kernels, cooked - 1/4 cup
- Red bell pepper, diced - 1/4 cup
- Avocado, diced - 1/2
- Cherry tomatoes, halved - 1/4 cup
- 1 tablespoon lime juice
- 1 tablespoon chopped cilantro
- To taste, add cumin, paprika, and chili powder.

Season with salt and pepper to taste.

### Instructions

Cooked quinoa, black beans, cooked corn kernels, chopped red bell pepper, diced avocado, and split cherry tomatoes should all be combined in a dish.

Squeeze lime juice over the mixture and top with cilantro.

Season to taste with cumin, paprika, chili powder, salt, and pepper.

Toss everything together until everything is fully integrated.

Serve refrigerated or at room temperature.

# DINNER RECIPES

## *Baked Teriyaki Salmon*

- Salmon fillets - 2
- Teriyaki sauce 1/4 cup
- Honey 1 tablespoon
- 1 teaspoon tamari (gluten-free soy sauce) or soy sauce
- Chopped garlic cloves - 2
- Grated ginger - 1 teaspoon

**Optional garnishes:** sesame seeds and chopped green onions

Season with salt and pepper to taste.

**Instructions**

Preheat the oven to 400 degrees F (200 degrees C).

Whisk together teriyaki sauce, honey, soy sauce or tamari, chopped garlic, grated ginger, salt, and pepper in a mixing bowl.

Place the salmon fillets in a baking dish.

Pour the teriyaki sauce mixture over the salmon, coating it well.

Marinate the salmon for 20-30 minutes in the refrigerator.

Bake the salmon for 12-15 minutes, or until it reaches the desired level of doneness, in a preheated oven.

To keep the salmon moist, baste it with the marinade many times during baking.

Remove the salmon from the oven and set aside for a few minutes to rest.

If preferred, garnish with sesame seeds and sliced green onions.

Serve immediately.

## *Thai Coconut Curry with Vegetables and Tofu*

**Ingredients**

- 8 ounces diced firm tofu
- 2 cups mixed veggies (including bell peppers, broccoli, and snap peas)
- 1 can (13.5 oz) coconut milk
- 2 teaspoons red curry paste
- 2 tablespoons soy sauce or tamari (gluten-free soy sauce)
- 1 tsp lime juice
- Minced garlic cloves - 2
- Grated ginger - 1 teaspoon
- Thai basil and sliced red chiles are optional garnishes.

Season with salt and pepper to taste.

**Instructions**

Warm the coconut milk in a large pan or wok over medium-high heat.

To the skillet, add the red curry paste, chopped garlic, grated ginger, salt, and pepper. Stir until well blended.

Cook the cubed tofu in the pan until it is gently browned.

Cook for 10 minutes, or until the vegetables are tender-crisp.

Pour in the lime juice and soy sauce or tamari. To coat the ingredients, stir them together.

Reduce the heat to low and allow the flavors to combine for a few minutes.

If necessary, adjust the seasoning.

If preferred, garnish with Thai basil leaves and sliced red chiles.

Thai coconut curry is best served with steamed rice or noodles.

Serve immediately.

## *Skillet with Turkey and Vegetables*

### Ingredients

- 8 ounces of ground turkey
- 1/2 cup chopped onion
- Garlic cloves, minced - 2
- 2 cups mixed veggies (zucchini, bell peppers, and carrots)
- Sauce with tomatoes 1 cup
- Olive oil 2 teaspoons
- Italian seasoning 1 teaspoon

Season with salt and pepper to taste.

### Instructions

Warm the olive oil in a large pan over medium heat.

To the skillet, add the chopped onion and minced garlic. Cook until the onion is transparent.

Cook until the ground turkey is browned and cooked thoroughly in the pan.

Cook for 10 minutes, or until the vegetables are tender-crisp.

Season the tomato sauce in the pan with Italian seasoning, salt, and pepper.

Stir everything together and let aside for a few minutes to allow the flavors to blend.

If necessary, adjust the seasoning.

Serve the turkey and veggie skillet with cooked rice or noodles.

Serve immediately.

## Lentil Curry

**Ingredients**

- Lentils - 1 cup
- Onion, diced - 1/2 cup
- Garlic cloves, minced - 2
- Ginger, grated - 1 teaspoon
- Curry powder - 1 tablespoon
- Turmeric - 1/2 teaspoon
- Cumin - 1/2 teaspoon
- Coriander - 1/2 teaspoon
- Coconut milk - 1 can (13.5 ounces)
- Vegetable broth - 1 cup
- Mixed vegetables (such as carrots, bell peppers, and peas) - 2 cups

- Olive oil - 2 tablespoons
- Fresh cilantro, chopped - for garnish

Salt and pepper to taste

**Instructions**

Remove any debris from the lentils by rinsing them under cool water.

Warm the olive oil in a big saucepan over medium heat.

Add diced onion, minced garlic, and grated ginger to the pot. Sauté until the onion becomes translucent.

Combine the curry powder, turmeric, cumin, and coriander in a mixing bowl. Cook for a minute until fragrant.

Add the rinsed lentils, coconut milk, vegetable broth, and mixed vegetables to the pot.

Bring the mixture to a boil, then reduce the heat to low and simmer for about 20-25 minutes or until the lentils are tender, stirring occasionally.

Season with salt and pepper to taste.

Serve the lentil stew with naan bread or steamed rice.

Garnish with fresh chopped cilantro.

Serve hot.

## *Zucchini Noodles with Turkey Meatballs*

### Ingredients

- Zucchini - 2
- Ground turkey - 8 ounces
- Onion, finely chopped - 1/4 cup
- Garlic cloves, minced - 2
- Fresh parsley, chopped - 2 tablespoons
- Egg - 1
- Almond flour or breadcrumbs - 1/4 cup
- Tomato sauce - 1 cup
- Olive oil - 2 tablespoons
- Italian seasoning - 1 teaspoon

Salt and pepper to taste

### Instructions

Spiralize or julienne peel the zucchini to make zucchini noodles (zoodles). Set aside.

In a bowl, combine ground turkey, finely chopped onion, minced garlic, chopped parsley, egg, almond flour or breadcrumbs, Italian seasoning, salt, and pepper. Mix well to combine.

Form the turkey mixture into small meatballs.

Warm the olive oil in a pan over medium heat. Cook until the meatballs are browned on both sides and cooked through in the pan.

Set the meatballs aside after removing them from the pan.

In the same skillet, add tomato sauce and bring it to a simmer.

Cook the zucchini noodles in the skillet for 2-3 minutes, or until they are soft.

Return the cooked meatballs to the skillet with the zucchini noodles.

Toss everything together until the meatballs and zucchini noodles are coated with tomato sauce.

Serve hot.

## *Shrimp Stir-Fry with Brown Rice*

### Ingredients

- Shrimp, peeled and deveined - 8 ounces
- Mixed vegetables (such as broccoli, snap peas, and carrots) - 2 cups
- Garlic cloves, minced - 2
- Ginger, grated - 1 teaspoon
- Low-sodium soy sauce or tamari (gluten-free soy sauce) - 2 tablespoons
- Sesame oil - 1 tablespoon

**Optional:** red pepper flakes for added heat

- Cooked brown rice - 2 cups

Salt and pepper to taste

## Instructions

In a large skillet or wok, heat sesame oil over medium-high heat.

Add minced garlic, grated ginger, and optional red pepper flakes to the skillet. Sauté for a minute until fragrant.

Add the shrimp to the skillet and stir-fry until they turn pink and are cooked through.

Set the shrimp aside after removing them from the skillet.

In the same skillet, stir-fry the mixed vegetables until they are tender-crisp.

Return the cooked shrimp and veggies to the skillet.

Add low-sodium soy sauce or tamari to the skillet and toss everything together.

Season with salt and pepper to taste.

Serve the shrimp stir-fry over brown rice that has been prepared.

Serve hot.

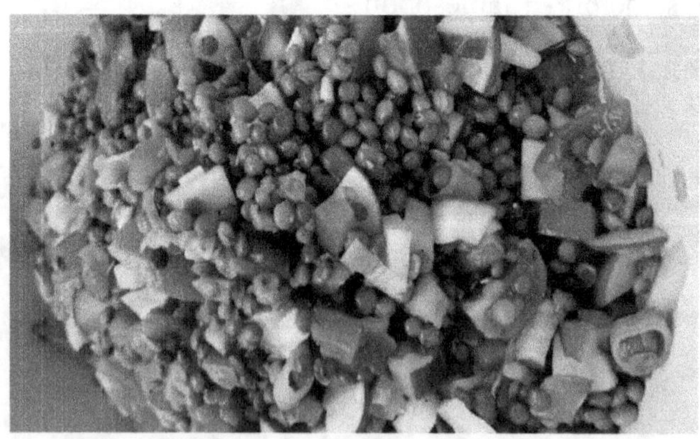

## *Mediterranean Grilled Chicken Skewers*

### Ingredients

- Chicken breast, cut into cubes - 2
- Red onion, cut into chunks - 1/2
- Cherry tomatoes - 10
- Zucchini, sliced - 1
- Bell peppers, cut into chunks - 1/2
- Olive oil - 2 tablespoons
- Lemon juice - 2 tablespoons
- Garlic cloves, minced - 2
- Dried oregano - 1 teaspoon

Salt and pepper to taste

### Instructions

Preheat the grill to medium-high heat.

In a bowl, whisk together olive oil, lemon juice, minced garlic, dried oregano, salt, and pepper to make the marinade.

Thread the chicken cubes, red onion chunks, cherry tomatoes, zucchini slices, and bell pepper chunks onto skewers.

Brush the marinade over the skewered ingredients, ensuring they are well-coated.

Grill the skewers for 10-12 minutes, flipping regularly, until the chicken is cooked through and the veggies are soft.

Remove the skewers from the grill and set aside for a few minutes to rest.

Serve hot.

## Baked Sweet Potato with Black Bean and Quinoa

**Ingredients**

- Sweet potatoes - 2 medium-sized
- Cooked quinoa - 1 cup
- 1 cup cooked and drained black beans
- Red onion, diced - 1/4 cup
- Bell peppers, diced - 1/4 cup
- Cilantro chopped - 2 tablespoons
- Lime juice - 2 tablespoons
- Olive oil - 1 tablespoon
- Cumin, paprika, and chili powder - to taste

Salt and pepper to taste

**Instructions**

Preheat the oven to 400°F (200°C).

Wash the sweet potatoes and pat them dry. With a fork, pierce each sweet potato many times.

Place the sweet potatoes on a baking sheet and bake in the preheated oven for about 45-60 minutes or until they are tender.

Prepare the filling while the sweet potatoes are baking. In a bowl, combine cooked quinoa, black beans, diced red onion, diced bell peppers, chopped cilantro, lime juice, olive oil, cumin, paprika, chili powder, salt, and pepper. Toss everything together.

Once the sweet potatoes are cooked, slice them lengthwise and gently mash the flesh with a fork.

Fill the sweet potato halves with the black bean and quinoa mixture.

Return the stuffed sweet potatoes to the oven for about 10-15 minutes to heat through.

Serve hot.

## Stir-Fried Beef with Vegetables

### Ingredients

- Beef steak (such as sirloin or flank steak) - 8 ounces, thinly sliced
- Mixed vegetables (such as broccoli, bell peppers, and carrots) - 2 cups, sliced
- 2 tablespoons soy sauce or tamari (gluten-free soy sauce)
- Sesame oil - 1 tablespoon
- Garlic cloves, minced - 2
- Ginger, grated - 1 teaspoon

**Optional:** red pepper flakes for added heat

Salt and pepper to taste

### Instructions

In a bowl, marinate the thinly sliced beef in soy sauce or tamari for about 10-15 minutes.

In a large skillet or wok, heat sesame oil over medium-high heat.

Add minced garlic, grated ginger, and optional red pepper flakes to the skillet. Sauté for a minute until fragrant.

Add the marinated beef to the skillet and stir-fry until it is cooked to your desired level of doneness.

Set the steak aside after removing it from the skillet.

In the same skillet, stir-fry the mixed vegetables until they are tender-crisp.

Return the cooked beef to the skillet with the vegetables and toss everything together.

Season with salt and pepper to taste.

Serve hot.

## Lemon Herb Roasted Chicken

### Ingredients

- Chicken thighs or breasts - 4 pieces
- Lemon - 1
- Fresh herbs (such as rosemary, thyme, or parsley) - a handful
- Garlic cloves - 4
- Olive oil - 2 tablespoons

Salt and pepper to taste

### Instructions

Preheat the oven to 425°F (220°C).

In a baking dish, place the chicken pieces.

Squeeze the lemon juice over the chicken.

Mince the garlic cloves and chop the fresh herbs. Sprinkle them over the chicken.

Drizzle the chicken with olive oil.

Season with salt and pepper.

Place the baking dish in the preheated oven and bake for about 30-35 minutes or until the chicken is cooked through and golden brown.

Serve hot.

# SNACKS

## Trail Mix with Nuts and Seeds

- Mixed nuts (such as almonds, walnuts, and cashews) - 1/4 cup
- Pumpkin seeds - 1 tablespoon
- Sunflower seeds - 1 tablespoon
- Dried cranberries or raisins - 1 tablespoon

**Optional:** sprinkle of cinnamon or nutmeg for added flavor

**Instructions**

In a small bowl, mix the mixed nuts, pumpkin seeds, sunflower seeds, and dried cranberries or raisins.

Add a sprinkle of cinnamon or nutmeg, if desired, for extra flavor.

To achieve uniform distribution, toss the ingredients together.

Transfer the trail mix to a resealable container for easy snacking on the go.

Enjoy a handful of the trail mix whenever you need a quick and nutritious snack.

# Roasted Chickpeas

## Ingredients

- 1 can (15 oz) drained and washed chickpeas (garbanzo beans)
- 1 tablespoon olive oil
- 1 teaspoon ground cumin
- 1/2 teaspoon smoked paprika
- 1/4 teaspoon garlic powder

Salt and pepper to taste

## Instructions

Preheat the oven to 400°F (200°C) and line a baking sheet with parchment paper.

Pat the chickpeas dry with a paper towel and remove any loose skins.

In a bowl, toss the chickpeas with olive oil, ground cumin, smoked paprika, garlic powder, salt, and pepper.

Spread the seasoned chickpeas on the baking sheet in a single layer.

Roast for 20-25 minutes, shaking the baking sheet halfway through to ensure even cooking, until the chickpeas are crispy and lightly browned.

# Baked Zucchini Fries

## Ingredients

- 2 medium zucchinis, cut into fries
- 1/4 cup almond flour
- 1/4 cup grated Parmesan cheese (optional, omit for dairy-free)
- 1 teaspoon paprika
- 1/2 teaspoon garlic powder
- Salt and pepper to taste
- 1 large egg, beaten (or egg substitute for egg-free version)

## Instructions

Preheat the oven to 425°F (220°C) and line a baking sheet with parchment paper.

In a shallow dish, mix almond flour, grated Parmesan cheese (if using), paprika, garlic powder, salt, and pepper.

Dip each zucchini fry into the beaten egg (or egg substitute) and then coat it with the almond flour mixture.

Place the coated zucchini fries on the baking sheet in a single layer.

Bake for 15-20 minutes or until the fries are crispy and golden brown.

## *Tuna Cucumber Bites*

### Ingredients

- 1 large cucumber
- 1 can (5 oz) tuna, drained
- 1-2 tablespoons mayonnaise or Greek yogurt
- 1 teaspoon Dijon mustard
- 1/4 teaspoon garlic powder
- Salt and pepper to taste
- Fresh dill or parsley for garnish

### Instructions

Slice the cucumber into rounds, about 1/2-inch thick.

In a bowl, mix the drained tuna, mayonnaise or Greek yogurt, Dijon mustard, garlic powder, salt, and pepper until well combined.

Place a spoonful of the tuna mixture on top of each cucumber slice.

Garnish with fresh dill or parsley for added flavor

## *Quinoa and Veggie Stuffed Mushrooms*

### Ingredients

- 10-12 large button mushrooms
- 1/2 cup cooked quinoa
- 1/4 cup finely chopped bell peppers
- 1/4 cup finely chopped zucchini
- 2 green onions, finely chopped
- 1 tablespoon olive oil
- 1/2 teaspoon dried oregano

- Salt and pepper to taste
- 1/4 cup grated Parmesan cheese (optional, omit for dairy-free)

**Instructions**

Preheat the oven to 375°F (190°C) and lightly grease a baking dish.

Remove the stems from the mushrooms and finely chop them.

In a skillet, heat olive oil over medium heat. Add chopped mushroom stems, bell peppers, zucchini, green onions, dried oregano, salt, and pepper. Sauté until vegetables are tender.

In a bowl, mix the cooked quinoa with the sautéed vegetables and optional Parmesan cheese.

Stuff each mushroom cap with the quinoa and vegetable mixture.

Place the stuffed mushrooms on the baking dish and bake for 15-20 minutes until the mushrooms are tender.

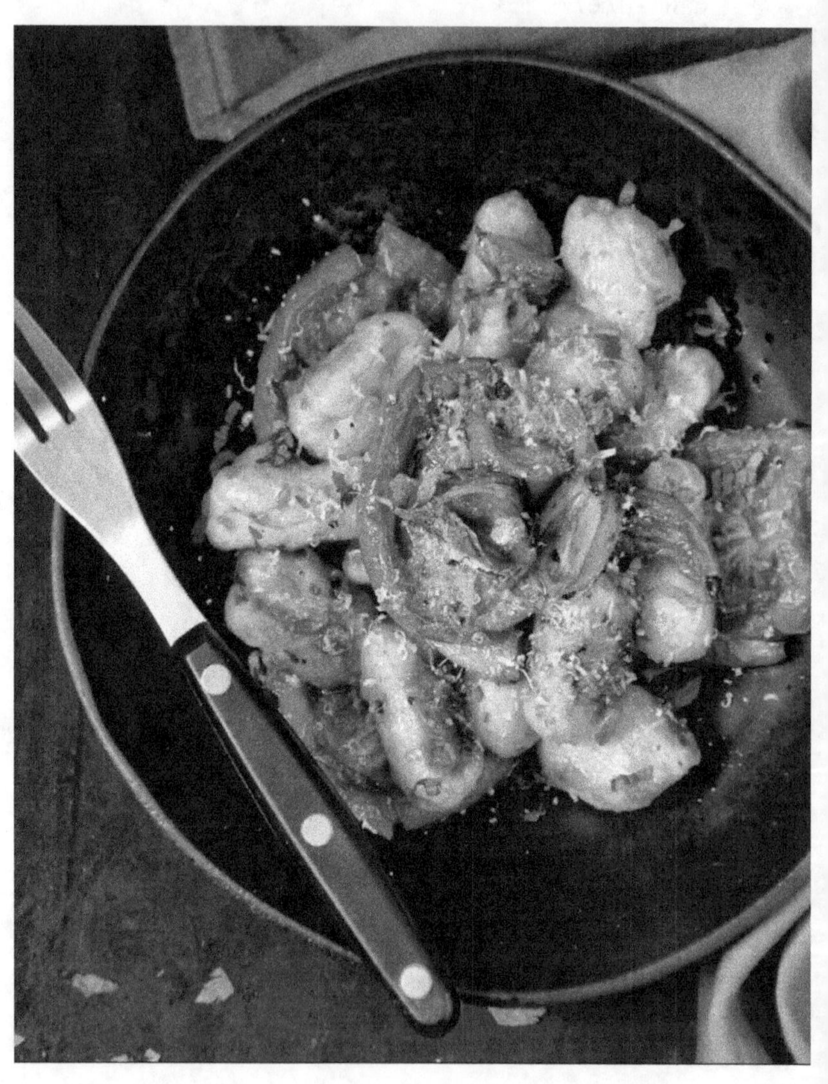

# DESSERTS

## *Baked Apple Slices with Cinnamon*

**Ingredients**

- 2-3 medium apples (use sweet varieties like Honeycrisp or Fuji)
- 1 tablespoon melted coconut oil or ghee (clarified butter)
- 1 teaspoon ground cinnamon

**Optional:** a drizzle of pure maple syrup or honey for added sweetness

**Instructions**

Preheat the oven to 375°F (190°C) and line a baking sheet with parchment paper.

Core the apples and slice them into thin rounds or wedges.

In a bowl, toss the apple slices with melted coconut oil or ghee, ground cinnamon, and optional maple syrup or honey.

Arrange the coated apple slices on the baking sheet in a single layer.

Bake for 15-20 minutes or until the apples are tender and lightly caramelized.

## *Coconut Vanilla Chia Popsicles*

**Ingredients**

- 1 can (13.5 oz) full-fat coconut milk
- 2 tablespoons chia seeds
- 1 tablespoon pure maple syrup or honey

- 1 teaspoon vanilla extract
- Fresh fruit slices (strawberries, mango, etc.) for added texture (optional)

**Instructions**

In a blender, combine coconut milk, chia seeds, maple syrup or honey, and vanilla extract. Blend until smooth.

If desired, add some fresh fruit slices into the mixture for added texture.

Pour the mixture into popsicle molds and insert popsicle sticks.

Freeze for at least 4 hours or until the popsicles are set.

To remove the popsicles from the molds, run warm water around the exterior of the molds for a few seconds to loosen the popsicles.

## Dark Chocolate-Covered Strawberries

**Ingredients**

- Fresh strawberries, washed and dried
- 1 cup dark chocolate chips (choose dairy-free if needed)

**Instructions**

Using parchment paper, line a baking sheet.

In a microwave-safe bowl or using a double boiler, melt the dark chocolate chips until smooth.

Dip each strawberry into the melted chocolate, covering about two-thirds of the berry.

Place the chocolate-covered strawberries on the parchment paper-lined baking sheet.

Refrigerate until the chocolate sets.

## *Almond Butter Banana Bites*

### Ingredients

- 2 ripe bananas, sliced into rounds
- 2 tablespoons almond butter (or any nut butter of choice)
- Unsweetened shredded coconut for rolling (optional)

### Instructions

Spread a small amount of almond butter on one side of each banana round.

Sandwich two banana rounds together with the almond butter sides facing each other.

**Optional:** Roll the almond butter banana bites in unsweetened shredded coconut for extra flavor and texture.

## *Baked Pears with Cinnamon and Walnuts*

### Ingredients

- 2 ripe pears, halved and cored
- 1 tablespoon melted coconut oil or ghee (clarified butter)
- 1 teaspoon ground cinnamon
- 2 tablespoons chopped walnuts

**Optional:** a drizzle of pure maple syrup or honey for added sweetness

## Instructions

Preheat the oven to 375°F (190°C) and line a baking sheet with parchment paper.

Place the pear halves on the baking sheet, cut side up.

Brush the melted coconut oil or ghee over the cut side of each pear half.

Sprinkle ground cinnamon over the pear halves and top with chopped walnuts.

**Optional:** Drizzle a small amount of pure maple syrup or honey over each pear half for added sweetness.

Bake for 20-25 minutes or until the pears are tender and lightly caramelized.

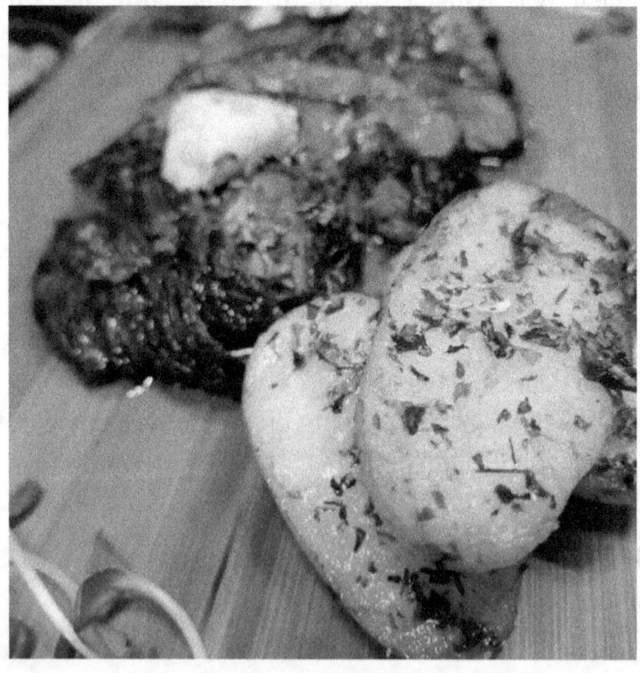

# CONCLUSION

Finally, this book has shed light on the complex nature of Hashimoto's disease, from its origins to the wide range of symptoms it produces. However, behind the difficulties is a light of hope and empowerment for those who read these pages.

We discovered the transformational power of conscious decisions as we investigated dietary and lifestyle changes to control Hashimoto's.

The dishes offered here not only tempt the taste senses, but they also serve as important aids in promoting general well-being.

Each meal can provide sustenance and vitality to the body, paving the path for a better and more balanced existence.

This book, however, goes beyond recipes to convey a message of self-empowerment and perseverance. We acquire agency over our health by taking responsibility of our eating, which fosters a sense of control and fresh resolve.

Each meal becomes a tremendous step toward better health and a reminder of the strength we possess.

As you close the book's last pages, I hope you will be inspired to live a life of nourishment, awareness, and empowerment.

Remember that you have the strength to conquer and prosper, whether you are suffering with Hashimoto's or any other challenge.

Allow this trip to serve as a reminder that with perseverance and a balanced approach, we can overcome even the most severe of obstacles.

May the wisdom learned from these pages serve as a springboard to a life full of energy, pleasure, and the awareness that, regardless of the odds, a meaningful and powerful life awaits those who dare to take responsibility for their destiny.

Allow this book to serve as your guide to discovering your route to a healthier, happier, and more vibrant existence.

**Would you like to check other books by this author? Or recommend it to your loved ones.**

DIABETIC DIET AFTER 50

THE ANTI-INFLAMMATORY DIET FOR BEGINNERS

RENAL DIET COOKBOOK FOR BEGINNERS

www.ingramcontent.com/pod-product-compliance
Lightning Source LLC
Chambersburg PA
CBHW060214260726

48658CB00005BA/2035